A HALF BUBBLE OUT OF PLUMB

LAUGHTER IS GOOD MEDICINE

BY:
WINSTON H. HUNT, P.A.

LIGHT SWITCH
PRESS

Published by:
Light Switch Press
PO Box 272847
Fort Collins, CO 80527
www.lightswitchpress.com

Copyright © 2016

ISBN: 978-1-944255-37-4

Printed in the United States of America

No part of this publication may be reproduced, stored in a retrieval system, or transmitted in any form or by any means – electronic, mechanical, digital photocopy, recording, or any other without the prior permission of the author.

All rights reserved solely by the author. The author guarantees all contents are original and do not infringe upon the legal rights of any other person or work. The views expressed in this book are not necessarily those of the publisher.

DEDICATION

This book is dedicated to all the health care providers, from housekeepers to physicians, who I met while working in the medical field.

I hope that those who are currently providing health care, along with patients, will appreciate that laughter does heal.

This book is especially dedicated to the many patients who unknowingly provided these memories and to my wife Debbie who helped edit and put up with me during the many hours of writing and rewriting this work. She has also put up with me for over forty-five years of marriage.

Special thanks go out to Scott Vasquez, my son-in-law, and Jennifer, my daughter, who typed and re-typed this work.

INDEX

Preface I
Before Diuretics 1
Don't Pant 3
A Near Miss Shooting 7
Pediatrics Not for Me 11
A Changed Person 13
The Longest Weekend 19
Dentures Please 21
Physician Assistant Education 23
Don't Lose Your Clamp 25
Where's the Patch? 31
Listing to the Right 37
A Pet Flying Squirrel 39
Too Many Showers 45
Where's The Phone? 49

PREFACE

"A Half Bubble Out of Plumb" is a collection of funny stories, memories and miracles that I remember while working in the medical field for approximately fifty years.

This journey started when I was almost 5 years old. Our family moved from New Jersey to Augusta, Georgia in 1953. Augusta was known for its' major golf tournament, a nearby nuclear bomb plant, Camp Gordon and the Medical College of Georgia. It was a segregated southern town located on the banks of the Savannah River which separated Georgia and South Carolina.

My father, Whitelaw, was the new Director of the city's University Hospital. He would direct it through desegregation and a growth phase spanning the next thirteen years. He died in December of 1966 after helping to see a $5-million-dollar hospital bond pass. The bond passage would help build a new University Hospital with 700 beds and a price tag nearing $22 million dollars at the time.

As part of his compensation package, a residence was provided for the family adjacent to the hospital. Living this close to a hospital sparked a desire in me and both my brothers to do something in the medical field. Whit Jr. and Wyman became hospital administrators while I worked my way up the ladder from ambulance attendant to Physician Assistant.

After my father died, I dropped out of college and began my almost five-decade journey in the medical field. I have compiled this series of short stories drawn from my experiences while working as an ambulance attendant, emergency room and nursing home orderly, Navy Corpsmen in Vietnam, pharmaceutical representative, college professor and Physician Assistant.

This book is not intended to serve in any way as a medical text. It is for your enjoyment only. Any references to diseases or treatments are offered in their simplest of terms as adjuncts to my stories and are not recommended for use other than clarification and entertainment.

I hope you will enjoy "A Half Bubble Out of Plumb" and that you will find laughter does have some healing property. You will also see in some of the stories where patients, students, co-workers and even myself were maybe a burger short of a happy meal, had an IQ of room temperature or were two bricks short of a load --- and, YES, a half bubble out of plumb.

BEFORE DIURETICS

The family packed up, in the summer of 1953, and headed south along US highway one. It was the beginning of a new life in a new state and city. I was turning five years old when we moved so that my father could become the Director of a hospital in Augusta, Georgia.

The hospital was located in the inner city section of Augusta, Georgia. A residence was provided on the hospital grounds for our family. It was a two story brick, four bed room structure with a couple of window air conditioners. It was located so close to the side of the hospital's Jennings Wing that I can remember lying in bed, listening to patients groaning, gasping for breath (dyspnea) and wondering what was wrong with them. Behind the house was a closed Children's Hospital (Wilhenford Hospital for Children) and the Doughty Nurse's Home which housed nursing students. In front of the house was hospital visitor parking. Several physician offices, a drug store and a small family owned grocery store were a mere stone's throw away. This combined with the Medical College on the west made it the hub of the Augusta Medical Community.

The hospital was like a city within a city. There were maintenance, engineering, laundry, carpentry and printing departments. We received our family calls and mail through the hospital. The only neighbors we had were the employees of the hospital.

As the years passed, I began to understand what was happening to the patients I had heard crying out, choking and gasping for breath on many long summer nights (there was no central air conditioning at that time). They most likely were suffering from a form of congestive heart failure (CHF) or pulmonary embolism (PE). This was before diuretics had been developed and many of these patients were drowning in their own body fluids. Their lungs were filling up making breathing extremely difficult. The loop diuretics of the furosemide class didn't come out until the mid-sixties. These water pills helped the kidneys clear excess fluid which made the patients breathing easier.

As the Director's son all doors seemed to be open to me so I began to nose around the various sections of the hospital. I started going to the Emergency

Room (ER) on weekends to see what was going on. Anytime there was a bad accident, shooting or something else big happening, I was there.

The private physicians took notice of my interest in medicine and started to let me follow them into treatment rooms. I would watch them suture wounds, perform CPR or whatever they were doing. I became pretty good at reading x-rays. By age fourteen I could point out fractures, tumors and even foreign bodies. I would help transport patients to the Operating Room (OR), X-ray or patient rooms for admission. The opportunity to learn over the ensuing years was great and exciting.

I especially enjoyed it when new ER Residents arrived (these were graduate physicians who wanted to specialize in Emergency medicine). I would show up and walk into a treatment room to see what was happening. This made some of the new residents uneasy and they would invariably ask someone who I was. Once they found out I was the Director's son the atmosphere often changed. Most of them also became willing to share with me what they were doing.

Eight hundred employees were involved with day-to-day operation of the hospital. They made up the Laboratory, Pharmacy, Pathology, X-Ray and other departments. The employees opened doors for me to learn all I could about their role in health care. I learned at a young age that there were no small positions in the delivery of health care.

I overheard my father share the following story with my mother one evening. An elderly patient had been admitted and he had given instructions not to be placed in a hot bath tub. He told some staff that for seventy years he had only bathed in spring water. He had been told by somebody not to take a hot bath and was passing this information on. The message didn't get passed down the line for some reason and he was placed in a hot tub. He soon became very agitated and died shortly thereafter. The hot water must have caused his blood vessels and organs to dilate and he sort of drowned in his own fluids. I learned an important lesson at an early age; listen to the patient.

My father died on December 22, 1966 at the age of fifty-three. My mother, Ruth, would remain a widow. My brothers, Whitelaw and Wyman, became hospital administrators while my sister, Cynthia, became a public school teacher. I dropped out of college, joined the local Naval Reserve unit with the full intention of becoming a corpsman.

DON'T PANT

I was given some family leave time before attending the Navy Hospital Corps School in Great Lakes, Illinois. Upon graduation from Corps School and while waiting for active duty orders, I took a couple of jobs to help keep my newly acquired corpsmen skills sharp. During my first job as an ambulance attendant, I learned another early lesson.

I was only nineteen when a call came in to pick up a pregnant lady for transport to the hospital. It was an extremely hot summer day when we got the call. Back then we were running Pontiac and Buick ambulances which were high topped station wagons and barely big enough to hold patients. They weren't even close to today's units, you know the ones with the big boxes attached to pickup truck frames.

The house was only about eight blocks away from the hospital. My driver was also new and both of us were a little apprehensive about the call. The house was the middle structure of three row houses known as the Three Sisters. They were located on Reynolds Street, just south of the levee and across from the TV station (the levee had been constructed in 1913 after the third flooding of the Savannah River in twenty-four years).

The call was to pick up a pregnant lady for transport to the hospital. Nothing was said about her being in labor. We were met by a young man who took us up the stairs to where his wife was. He appeared very nervous and as we entered her room it became obvious why he was so nervous. His wife was sitting on the bed nearly nude and screaming at the top of her voice. This was their first baby and she was definitely in labor. My driver and I looked at each other, assessed the scene, and began to load her onto a stretcher. We had to carry her down three stories to our unit. Hospital Corps School had not taught me how to deliver babies, so time was critical.

I was in the back trying to calm her down and suggested she start panting. I thought this would help her to relax. My next lesson came quickly. As we crossed the railroad tracks by the Coca-Cola building on Thirteen Street, she yelled out really loudly. I asked her what happened and she yelled "I just wet myself all over". I immediately told her to stop panting and told my driver to step on it. He radioed the ER and let them know we were about three blocks out. When we pulled up to the hospital we went straight through the ER and got on the elevator heading to Labor and Delivery (L & D). She delivered as we got off the elevator. The lesson I learned was don't tell a pregnant lady in labor to pant while you're in the back of an ambulance. I decided right then and there to let dogs and penguins do the panting to cool themselves. Talk about the blind leading the blind.

On another call we were sent up Broad Street to a housing authority complex located near the textile mill and canal. A patient was to be transported to the Cleckley Psychiatric Building for direct admission. The building was named for Hervey Cleckley who wrote, "Mask of Sanity." The book later became the movie "The Three Faces of Eve."

When we arrived, we were greeted by a seventy-year-old man sitting on his bed wielding a baseball bat. He threatened us shouting, "You are not going to take me anywhere." We looked for some patient restraints and couldn't find any, so we called for backup and requested the restraints. No one had told us how far out there this man was. When the unit arrived we decided to jump him on the count of three and put the restraints on. We jumped him on the count of three and he almost whipped the four of us before we could get him restrained. He fought me all the way to the Cleckley building which seemed like a hundred miles away. I learned right then that a psychiatric patient can become very strong when agitated no matter how old they are.

It was a typical hot, humid, gnat-spitting summer day when a call came in to send all our units to an airplane accident near Aiken, SC. The accident was somewhere between Clearwater and Aiken and involved a large commercial airplane.

Well, we jumped into our two units and headed across the Gordon Highway bridge into South Carolina. We took the Old Augusta Highway out of Clearwater toward Bath and Langley, SC, with our sirens blazing and pedals to the metal.

As we went through the villages, residents began to file in behind us to see what all the excitement was about. We were, after all, disturbing an otherwise quiet day in the valley. These were good decent people from textile mill families living along Horse Creek. Horse Creek, a tributary of the Savannah River, supplied water power for the early industries in the area. Textile mills were located along its' path as well as a pottery works in Vaucluse and a paper mill at one time in Bath. Most of the resident's homes had been built by these early textile mills and resembled row houses. I believe the area is called Midland Valley now. As we got closer to Aiken, a South Carolina Highway Patrol car passed us with lights and siren on. We knew we were headed for something big because we now had a police escort. We were led a very short distance before the patrol car pulled us over. The trooper wanted to know where we were going in such a hurry.

The trooper was wearing a straw hat, looked thirty something and was very upset with us. We told him about the call and airplane crash. He jumped back in his car and led us forward. He stopped us again a few more miles down the road. By this time, we kind of knew something was up and that we might be in trouble. Quite a procession of cars and pick-ups had filed in behind us by now. The trooper got out of his car and informed us that he had been on the radio and that he couldn't find an airplane crash or an accident of any kind within fifty miles of Aiken. The locals began getting out of their vehicles and were becoming very upset at us for disturbing their day and putting lives at risk driving so fast with the sirens on. They began to shout at us, telling us we had no call to be driving the way we did. The trooper suggested we get into our units, head over to US Highway One and get the heck back to Augusta as quietly as we could.

Within minutes of returning to our station, the calls began to come in from the mayors of the towns we had blown through. Letters would follow over the next few days. The SC State Patrol even called and respectfully requested that we confirm any future request for assistance with them before crossing the river again. Our owners put a big second on this and to my knowledge we never crossed the Savannah again.

A NEAR MISS SHOOTING

I decided to get out of the ambulance attendant business and became an ER orderly at University Hospital. One afternoon a young girl was brought in by her mother complaining of a stomach ache. While being examined, she delivered a full-term baby. She immediately got off the exam table and ran out of the ER yelling that we were trying to pass a baby off on her. The mother was running behind her shouting that she only brought her daughter in for a stomach ache, not a baby. They were both running through the parking lot with security in hot pursuit. It was quite a sight to see them running in circles and hysterically shouting, with hands flying all over the place, that it wasn't her baby.

One Saturday night, an elderly man was being transferred by ambulance to the ER with a gunshot wound (GSW) to the head. We setup a treatment room to receive him and put the Operating Room (OR) on standby. When the patient arrived he was fully conscious and able to tell us what had happened.

He was an unshaven elderly man with gray hair who appeared bent over some. He looked much older than his stated seventy years. He told us he lived in the country in a three-room wooden one-story house. There was no air conditioning or bathroom. The outhouse was in back and down-wind from the prevailing winds. He said he often sat on the porch at night to cool down. That night his dog would not stop barking.

"My old dog just wouldn't shut up barking at some fool rabbit, possum or something. I went inside to get my 22 caliber hand gun to shoot him if he wouldn't stop barking. I went outside and shot at him but the gun didn't go off. I fired two more times and nothing happened. I put the gun to my head, pulled the trigger and the dang thing fired." True story!

X-rays confirmed a bullet had entered one side of his head and had travelled between the skin and skull before stopping on the other side. The ER resident made a small incision in the skin and the bullet just popped out. A dressing as applied and he was as good as new. Before he left, the old man added, "When I get out from here I'm going to have to get new bullets." There were some of us who thought this was a miracle.

It seemed to always occur in the wee hours of the morning, street people would come to the ER to escape the elements. They would have various complaints to keep them out of the cold or rain. "I can't pee" was the most frequent problem. They knew it could be hours before a urinalysis would be performed at that time of the morning and they might not have to sleep under the bridge if we were busy.

One night I was having an extra difficult time obtaining a urine specimen from one of these street people. I asked my ER nurse if she had any tricks up her sleeves which might speed up the collection process. She was a seasoned nurse and suggested I try the following. Get the largest Foley catheter you can find and dangle it when you enter the treatment room. The patient should ask what is that and what are you going to do with it?

Tell him that you're going to put it (the catheter) into his bladder, through his thing, if he can't void (pee) in the next few minutes. Then leave the room with the patient holding a specimen cup and looking at the catheter and see how long it takes before he gives you a specimen. Guess what? When I returned in a few minutes, he had a full specimen cup for me to take to the laboratory. What a miracle. From then on, no one was going to stay in the ER all morning waiting to void on my shift especially when the beds were needed for true emergencies.

One night we were notified that a badly burned patient was in route from an accident on one of the bridges crossing the Savannah River. He had been in a head on collision and his car had burst into flames. He was also on fire and apparently made the decision to jump into the river in an attempt to put the flames out. He landed on the bank instead. He was severely burned and unfortunately didn't survive.

Another incident occurred when our receptionist yelled for help just before fainting to the floor. She had looked up to see a man standing in front of her with a screwdriver sticking out of his forehead. We learned he had been working on his car when a screwdriver fell down striking the engine fan and then ricocheted into his head. He had walked over six blocks in the heat to the ER with a screwdriver embedded to the handle in his forehead.

X-rays confirmed a six-inch screwdriver was in the middle of his head between the two hemispheres and that no damage had occurred to his brain. If the screwdriver had been a centimeter (or a fraction of an inch) on either side of center, it could have been a different ending to this story. The screwdriver was simply pulled out. Follow-up X-Rays revealed no brain swelling or bleeding and he walked out of the ER good as new. Some considered this a miracle.

My orders for active duty arrived and I was off to a Naval Air Station in Argentia, Newfoundland.

PEDIATRICS NOT FOR ME

I didn't know where Newfoundland was, so I got an atlas out and looked it up. Newfoundland is a Canadian province/island located way up on the Atlantic side of Nova Scotia, Canada. There was a Naval Air Station, that had a medical dispensary, located in Argentia which closed in 1994. Canada, Britain and the US all had bases in Newfoundland at one time or other. These facilities served as refueling and stop overs for flights to and from Europe during WWII.

I took off from an Air Force base in New Jersey headed for Argentia. It was a beautiful day in New Jersey but we landed in a snow storm. I thought, Great! I'm a Southern boy stationed here for the next two years!

Newfoundland turned out to be a pretty nice place after all. The zero-degree weather didn't feel like zero because of very low humidity. There were lakes, rolling hills and what looked like Christmas trees everywhere. The capital of Newfoundland is St. John's. There was a Holiday Inn which took my Gulf credit card so I stayed there often on weekends. I met a nice girl (Newf) and learned the Newfoundland stomp which is like a polka only with heavy stomps on the down beats. I got a Newfoundland driver's license and purchased an old car on base to commute back and forth to St. John's.

The dispensary was only one story, made of wood and painted white, of course. It wasn't a very big place and our quarters were partitioned rooms located in one of the wings. The staff was mainly reserves like myself and pretty laid back. On weekends we could get up and cook our own breakfast.

As fate would have it, my arrival coincided with the last big snow storm some nine months earlier. I was assigned to the new born nursery. While on duty one night, six babies were born. I was responsible for weighing, measuring, foot printing, bathing and feeding each one. The nursery was maintained at about ninety degrees. This quickly became one of my longest shifts. My nurse sat on her duff and never once offered any assistance. This wasn't the first time she hadn't offered to help. I knew a little about how to handle nurses from my ER days but military nurses are a different breed. I wouldn't win any show down with her. After the morning feedings, I went to see the base executive officer to let him know what I thought about the situation. I couldn't work with someone who wouldn't work with me. I told him I wanted to be a physician one day, just not a pediatrician. There just wasn't the excitement or learning potential here that I needed.

The exec heard my plea and told me the only way I was going to get my orders changed was to volunteer for Vietnam, so I did! During the next few weeks, I learned that one of the corpsmen who was sent to Vietnam, a month earlier, had been killed. I immediately started running laps around the dispensary and praying a lot.

Some weeks later, the exec called me to his office with my new orders. I was to report to the USS Repose-AH-16 in DaNang, South Vietnam. This was a hospital ship stationed in the combat waters off the Vietnam coast. My prayers had been answered and I was off on my next adventure. A journey my brother Wyman would later say changed my life.

A CHANGED PERSON

I will never forget the long flight aboard a Flying Tiger Airways jet from Los Angeles to Anchorage, Alaska and on into DaNang. The flight started off with everyone excited about where they were going. The closer we got to Nam, the quieter it got. Each passenger seemed to be reflecting on an uncertain future. Who was going to come back?

I would like to first give a brief background on the Hospital Ship Repose. The following ship's statistics come from either the Departure Ceremony pamphlet we received 14 March 1970 or the Repose Year Book 1969-1970.

"The USS Repose AH was first commissioned on 26 May 1945 and assigned to the U.S. Pacific fleet 14 July 1945. She was a hospital ship and saw duty in the North China Sea over the next two years. She was decommissioned once and reactivated on 16 October 1965. She arrived in Vietnam on 14 February 1966....

The Repose was painted all white and had red crosses on her sides, in accordance with the Geneva Convention. She was stationed off the Vietnam shore near the sites of the heaviest battles with expected high casualties. Helicopters would transport wounded directly from the battles to the ship. She sailed from DaNang to the Demilitarized Zone (17th parallel), receiving casualties....

Ship statistics show she had a bed capacity of 721 with 560 operating beds in the hospital. She had 19 line/supply officers, 24 medical officers, 3 dental officers, 29 Nurse Corps officers, 7 medical service corps officers, 290 ship crew, 246 hospital corpsmen and 7 dental technicians....

On 30 January 1967, she performed the 3000th consecutive successful helicopter landing. On March, she marked the 2000th surgical operation in Vietnam. USS Repose marked her 9000th safe helo landing on 14 November 1968 and her 10,000th helo landing on 27 January 1969. By the end of October 1969, Repose compiled these impressive statistics. After her 44th consecutive month in Vietnamese waters, she admitted a total of 22,610 patients of whom 8,493 were wounded in action....

Besides American service and civilian personnel, those treated included Vietnamese civilians and military, Thai, Filipino, Chinese, Korean and French personnel....

From 16 February 1966, when Repose arrived in Vietnam, through 10 March 1970, more than 24,000 patients had been admitted for in-patient care. Of this number, more than 9,000 (37%) were battle casualties. In addition, 37,000 out-patients had been seen and treated."

You can think of her as you would any of the level one trauma centers located throughout your state. These centers receive severely injured and sick patients from surrounding counties via life support helicopters mainly. The only difference is the Repose was on water sailing near the sites of heaviest battles and receiving virtually all her casualties from the combat zones via helicopters. We were so close to combat at times, you could hear the choppers taking off in route to the ship.

Corpsmen, like myself, were assigned to various duties throughout the hospital. Some worked in the intensive care unit, others in the operating room, while still others worked on the medical/surgical wards. Some were assigned to triage the helicopter casualties. I became a changed person. Looking down at quadruple amputees, about your own age, will have that effect on you. Ironically, almost to a man, they would look up at you and ask if they still had their thing.

During one shift, I was helping to transfer a patient from his stretcher onto an x-ray table when his leg came off in my hands. The only thing I could think of was to place the only leg he had come on board with back on the stretcher while continuing to put him on the x-ray table. This really hit home a few hours later.

Besides the Repose, two other hospital ships operated in the waters off Vietnam. Germany had the "Helgoland" which arrived in 1966. Her final harbor was the city of DaNang where only civilians were treated on board, no soldiers. When she left port we knew DaNang or the immediate area around DaNang was going to be hit. The locals who she treated didn't want anything to happen to her. We learned to leave port when she left. The USS Sanctuary, AH-17, arrived in April of 1967 to help with the increasing workload of combat casualties.

As unpopular as the war was, I would be doing a disservice by not mentioning those who supported our efforts. Several USO groups along with various bands touring Nam came on board to raise morale and make people laugh. Miss America participants and Playboy playmates brightened many a day. It seemed a lot of people realized what Bob Hope knew all along, that laughter was good medicine.

As I mentioned, it wasn't all work and no play aboard the Repose. There were sun decks, movies, a soda fountain and lounges where recuperating patients and crew hung out. There were beach parties on Qua Viet beach, volleyball, pickup basketball games and shuffle board games twenty-four seven. Every couple of months we sailed to Subic Bay, in the Philippines, to off-load and replenish supplies. Several crew members looked forward to seeing their Olongapo sweethearts. Others, like myself, saw this as an opportunity to travel and see the country.

Four of us set off for Manila during one of these Subic Bay replenishment visits. Manila is the capital city and we thought it would be cool to see it. We traveled by bus through the various provinces between Subic Bay and Manila. It was a hot and dusty ride because the bus had no air conditioning. It was loaded with local Philippine natives carrying goods to Manila for sale it seemed. Most were elderly women staring quietly out the open windows. Many of them were probably my age when WWII invaded their pristine islands. Now they carried baskets of vegetables, eggs, chickens and such to market. They looked like they were still trying to dig themselves out of the ravages of WWII.

At one point, we were boarded by some local militia. They had weapons and looked very imposing as they walked through the bus searching for possible rebels and questioning passengers. We wondered what they would do to anyone not answering them correctly. We also wondered if we would be taken off as spies and decided to smile a lot. The armed militia left the bus without incident. It reminded us just how much we take for granted our freedom of movement in America. As we moved on toward Manila, I saw a John Deere tractor plowing a nearby field.

There was a marked contrast from the country to when we entered Manila. We checked into an internationally known hotel that was just as modern as any found in Atlanta. It had the biggest chandelier I had ever seen hanging in the lobby. Our rooms were clean and had all the creature comforts of home.

Walking through the city, we saw the famous Philippines jeepneys. Jeepneys are the most popular means of public transportation in the Philippines. They are known for their crowded seating and brightly colored decorations. They were originally made from the jeeps left over from World War II. The Jeepneys were everywhere, packed full of locals and tourists. You couldn't miss them as they bussed through the streets with people hanging off of them. They sort of reminded me of the hippie peace-love buses in California. The Partridge family bus also comes pretty close because of its size and bright colors.

There is a special kind of sea snake unique to the waters of Vietnam. It is so venomous that if bitten you might have just enough time to say "Oh s..t!" before dying. They would float by our ship at night attracted to the lights which lit up our Red Crosses. We used slingshots and anything not tied down to try and hit them as they floated by. You could hear shouting when someone got one.

The following comes from a message our Captain sent to the Captain of the Sanctuary on 17 February 1970. "USS Repose hereby formally challenges USS Sanctuary to a one-hour drag race from a ten knot rolling start, to be held at Thunder Beach race track on or about 1 March after your return from bottom cleaning, face lifting and transplant surgery at SRF Medical Center, Subic....

All current safe engineering practices will be strictly adhered to. The use of ski wax, rigging of sails and the flying of nurse's laundry will not be allowed....

Repose additionally challenges Sanctuary to a lifeboat and/or whaleboat race with nurses as coxswain to start at Danit heads." I believe we won in a close finish.

The Repose left Vietnam to sail home for Decommissioning. Our return home was an adventure all its own. We returned via Subic Bay, Hong Kong, Osaka (Japan), Pearl Harbor and under the Golden Gate Bridge in San Francisco.

We spent two weeks in Hong Kong where I was able to pick up a guidebook compliments of the Hong Kong Hilton. This came in very handy while traversing streets crammed with millions of people. I took the Peak Tram cable car up to see a spectacular view of Hong Kong and the harbor far below. The harbor is surrounded by mountains, steep, rugged, treeless which made Hong Kong look very impressive from our ship's deck. The lights of Hong Kong were equally as beautiful reflecting off the water. This was in marked contrast to what I saw while walking the streets during the day, where poverty was seen everywhere. Clothes were hung between buildings. People were hanging out windows trying to cool themselves while others were living and cooking meals in the gutters.

Another not so pretty site were the Junk boats that traveled between ships in the harbor picking up left overs tossed from the sides of anchored vessels. Entire families lived aboard these once valued boats and you could see them cooking on the decks. It was time to move on so we lifted anchor to sail for Osaka, Japan.

While in Osaka, Japan, several of us took the time to visit Expo '70. The Exposition was a wonderful way for man to display his progress in science and technology. There were 85 pavilions to tour from all over the world. We only had a few hours, but managed to see about 10 exhibits. We wouldn't have seen that many if not for the wonderful way we were treated. Everywhere we went, we were put at the head of the line. The Japanese treated us like honored guests. Many wanted to take a picture of us in uniform. They were always bowing to us.

We sailed from Osaka, Japan to Pearl Harbor where we were also greeted as heroes. A Navy band was playing as we docked and the USO put on a luau as part of our decommissioning ceremonies. A few of us rented a car and drove all around the island. After a couple of weeks in Hawaii, we departed for San Francisco and Oakland, California.

Before we left Oakland to return to our homes we were told to take off our uniforms. Traveling in our civilian clothes was safer than in uniforms. If you didn't know it, Vietnam was a very unpopular war. Despite the unpopularity of the war, I feel proud of the services provided by the medical staff and ship's crew for the care the casualties received. Many a young man came home thanks to this combined effort. "Hooyah"!

I remained in the Naval Reserves for another couple of years which provided several funny incidents and fond memories.

THE LONGEST WEEKEND

As I previously mentioned, after returning from Vietnam I still had several years left in the Navy Reserves. Our unit would drill one weekend a month and each year we would spend two weeks on active duty. I had to plan my school and work around the active duty weeks and weekend drills.

I once spent two weeks in Pensacola, Florida filing x-rays at the Naval Air Station. During my off hours I would head to Fort Walton Beach, on the Gulf Coast, to check out the scenery. Another two weeks was spent in Charleston, South Carolina serving as an ambulance attendant and visiting some of the establishments along the strip.

One evening, while in Charleston, a few of us went to eat and have some cool ones. While seated at our table, we couldn't help but notice a lady at the next table. She was flopping her elbows against the side of her chest like a baby chicken. Every time her elbows hit her side her breast would grow bigger. I'm not kidding! She would hit the right side, with her elbow, and her right breast would enlarge. She would hit the left side, with her elbow, and her left breast would enlarge. When she hit her side with both elbows, both breast would inflate. The people at her table were having a time watching her, as were we. All of a sudden, the lady began to laugh. She was looking at a man at a table next to hers when he began knocking his knees together.

I signed up for a weekend cruise out of Charleston, SC on a submarine. I had never been aboard one so when the opportunity afforded itself, I jumped on it. This would turn out to be one of my longest weekends. The submarine was in Charleston for some crew rest and relaxation (R&R). Most of her regular crew were off so she was manned by reservists like myself. I learned quickly that submarine duty was not for me. I was six three, about two hundred twenty pounds and wore size twelve shoes. The ladder rungs were too small and the bunks too short. There wasn't enough room for me to stand straight up. Submarines ride smoother when submerged, so by the time we floated out of the harbor most of the crew was experiencing some form of motion sickness. Remember the crew was mainly composed of reservists and we were bobbing on the surface like a fishing bob. I was doing pretty good; after all, I had just crossed the Pacific on the Repose and even rode her through a typhoon.

The submarine was way smaller than the Repose and ran smoothly only when submerged. I got to go up into the conning tower which reminded me of some of the WWII movies I had seen. As I looked through the periscope I imagined I was looking at a German U-boat. This sub was cramped, dark, smelled and had poor air circulation. I had a nightmare the first night out and awoke in a cold sweat after just having fought off some sea monsters.

We developed an oil leak which meant we would have to remain top side until a tender arrived to refuel us. Great! Here we were bobbing on the surface and getting sicker all the time. While standing watch, the second night, the Captain came past me pale as a sheet. This along with the stench in the air finally got to me. The entire crew, including myself was praying for dry land where nothing moved to bring an end to this LONG weekend.

DENTURES PLEASE

I arrived home during the 1970 Augusta riots. It was a very unsettled time in Augusta's history. A mentally handicapped teenager was found dead in his cell after being arrested, apparently beaten by a fellow inmate. James Brown came home to help calm the situation because six people had been killed and about sixty injured during the ensuing day. Some three hundred people were arrested and several people went missing during this time.

My next adventure was to enroll in Augusta College (AC) and begin working as an orderly in the Georgia War Veterans Nursing Home, better known as the Blue Goose. I worked the eleven-to-seven am shift for the next two years while attending AC. I would get off the night shift at seven am and head for the Krispy Cream on Walton Way for breakfast. My first class began around eight am and I would continue classes until about three pm. I used my GI Bill, Navy Reserve pay and orderly pay to purchase a mobile home. I met my wife, Debbie, at AC and never looked back.

I must confess that college and I didn't get along very well at first. I just couldn't get it through my thick head that being able to tell the difference between a flute and a piccolo (Humanities 101) had anything to do with this life. Heck, I had just returned from Vietnam and traveled through much of Southeast Asia. I had visited a World's Fair, crossed the Equator, International Date Line and the Pacific Ocean.

One of my memories from the Blue Goose days happened early one morning, before I got off. Two residents began cussing, yelling and swinging at each other while sitting in their wheelchairs. They were in their late eighties, and it turned into a pretty good fight. We found out that someone had switched their dentures and they were trying to get them back. It looked like two old bucks clashing.

About this time my brother Wyman called me for some help. He was the Administrator in a nearby county hospital and was short of staff one New Year's Eve. He needed help covering the eleven pm to seven am shift. Since I had some healthcare experience he called on me to help. During the shift, a wreck victim came in who required surgery. The local surgeon asked if I wanted to assist him. He had been a Navy Surgeon and knew I was a Navy Reserve corpsman just back from Vietnam. During the surgery he informed me that he was going to be leaving the hospital to become the Director of the first Physician Assistant Program at the Medical College of Georgia. He thought I should apply and that I would have a good shot getting accepted. This was the beginning of another adventure. Thank you, Brother Wyman!

PHYSICIAN ASSISTANT EDUCATION

The Physician Assistant Program at the Medical College of Georgia would be accepting twenty students into the first class. Some of these students would have BS degrees, others two years of college and others no college at all. Those with no college would have clinical experience as EMT, military corpsmen, nursing assistants and so forth. This cross section would help develop future curriculum. I had enough credit hours from my three years at Augusta College and clinical experience which improved my chances. I was fortunate to be selected for the first class.

Physician Assistants (PA's) are trained academically and clinically to undertake many routine tasks traditionally performed by physicians. They can diagnose, treat and write prescriptions under the supervision of a physician. Training is divided between classroom lectures and clinical (hands on) experiences over two years. The training is similar to that given medical students. I immediately found myself overwhelmed with the likes of Biochemistry, Anatomy, Physiology and Pharmacology classes taught by the medical school professors. They were not going to change their lectures to suit us because many saw our profession as a conflict of interest. We were going to take jobs away from their ranks. Thank goodness I was a hands on learner, and with the help of classmates I was able to hang in there. I would help those that had no clinical experience and in return they would help me with the classroom courses. There was a lot of weekend tutoring going on.

We spent the last year doing rotations in Internal Medicine, Surgery, Family Medicine, Pediatrics, Emergency Medicine, Mental Health and a couple of electives in disciplines we wanted to learn more about. There was a lot of Mental Health training offered at the Georgia Regional Hospital and VA Hospital. Remember we were a new breed of health care provider and many physicians thought we were going to take jobs away from the medical school graduates. They were reluctant to help us. Upon graduation most colleges awarded a Bachelor of Science Degree. Now most award Master Degrees.

One of my electives was in Thoracic Surgery. I was able to observe open heart surgery procedures and learn how the open heart bypass machine functioned. My preceptor had moved from Walter Reed Hospital to Augusta to join a vascular surgery practice working out of University Hospital. He had been a MASH surgeon in Korea, and we hit it off right away. As a sidebar, on August 9, 1966 the first open heart surgery ever performed aboard a ship using cardio-pulmonary by-pass was successfully performed on a 13-year-old Vietnamese girl aboard the USS Repose, my old hospital ship. What a small world!

I spent my last elective rotation in Family Medicine with a physician who had a fascinating life story. He had dropped out of college to join the military during WWII. When he returned to Kentucky, he entered an accelerated General Medicine Program at the University of Kentucky. There was a shortage of physicians after WWII and programs like this were popping up in an effort to turn out more physicians to meet demands. This was very similar to the increase in MEDIX and Physician Assistant programs which sprang up after Korea and Vietnam when another physician shortage developed. There were thousands of military corpsmen ready to receive additional training and step up to the plate. During the end of this elective, my preceptor offered me a job and boy was I ready.

DON'T LOSE YOUR CLAMP

Thomson, Georgia is located about thirty miles west of Augusta. I had accepted a job there during my elective in Family Medicine because it qualified as a medically underserved area in Georgia. This was important since I had received a state scholarship and had agreed to work two years for every year of PA training in a designated medically underserved area of the state. It was payback time.

Dr. T was a Family Physician, OB-GYN and General Surgeon all rolled into one. He had a white crew cut that a B-52 could land on, and he always wore a bow tie. He loved his family, church, medical practice, golf and Cadillacs. The next five years were filled with many good memories and funny stories.

One day I was seeing an elderly lady for her regular checkup. She was the typical All-American grandmother. Her hair was pearl white, she was petite, polite and appreciated the care she was receiving. During the exam, she wanted to know if I could remove a growth on her face. I said I would be glad to and I asked her to lie down. While she was lying down, her wig fell off. This shocked me and embarrassed her. I had never seen a bald-headed lady before and started to chuckle. I left the room and tried not to lose it in front of her. Dr. T came out of a room and asked me what was so funny. We went into our lab area and I told him what had happened. I composed myself and went back into the room and removed the growth. Later that day Dr. T told me about an unexpected time he had in an ER once.

One evening he was on call at an ER, in Kentucky, when a lady brought in her daughter. The daughter was having a seizure and her mother was freaking out. The daughter was placed on a ER table and Dr. T injected her with some medication to stop the seizure. Well the girl stopped breathing! Her mother noticed this and started yelling, "She's not breathing." Dr. T looked at the mother and replied, "Well, she's not having any more seizures, is she?" The mother agreed and thanked him for stopping the seizures while the nurse escorted her out of the room. He said that, "If I had not kept calm during all this, I would have ended up treating two people instead of one." The girl was revived and all ended well. The point he was trying to make was to keep doing what you were trained to do when confronted by the unexpected and don't let the patient know anything differently.

I learned a lot from Dr. T as the years passed. He told me many stories of when he first started his practice in Kentucky. One day he was called to deliver a baby in a patient's home. He had to go way up into the mountains to get to her home. He traveled up a winding narrow dirt road, in his Buick, until the road literally ended in her front yard. It was so narrow by then that he couldn't even turn his car around. "I just left it there". Sometime later after the delivery he left the house and saw the Buick was turned around and headed down the mountain. "Somebody must have picked it up and turned it around because I had the keys in my pocket. I never heard or saw anything during this time to suggest anything else."

He told me about a man named Johnny who had had his hand smashed in an accident. He came into the office with this awfully mangled hand. Dr. T looked at it and told Johnny he would have to send him to Lexington where the hand would probably be cut off. "It was too badly mangled." Well, that was Johnny's brown bag hand and he started to beg Dr. T not to send him to Lexington. "You can save it", he pleaded. Dr. T agreed to try and save it and proceeded to do what he could. Later on, Johnny was going all around the town showing off his healing, yet still mangled hand to everyone. He was so happy that he hadn't lost it and was giving praise to Dr. T. "Doctor T did this", he shouted while proudly showing everyone the mangled hand. Dr. T saw and heard Johnny's shouts of joy and went up to him and told him, "Shut up fool I'm trying to start a practice here!" Old Johnny was about a half bubble out of plumb.

A young man came in for a scheduled vasectomy. I would be assisting Dr. T with this minor surgical procedure. The patient was nervous, as expected, and uncertain he had made the right decision. I prepped him and Dr. T came in to start the procedure. It was during this minor surgery that I learned another valuable lesson.

The surgery was pretty straight forward; find the sperm cords, clamp the cords, cut a wedge out between them and tie off the ends. Remove the clamps and, Bingo, it's over. Things were going along swimmingly until I heard Dr. T say, "Oh-Oh". The clamp on one of the cords had come off. The already nervous patient heard Dr. T's "Oh-Oh" and asked if everything was Ok. I remembered his previous lesson to continue to do what you were trained to do when the unexpected occurs, and don't let the patient know anything is wrong. Dr. T assured the young man everything was Ok and under control. He began to probe for the unclamped cord and the patient was beginning to squirm. "It feels like you're digging clear up to my belly button", he said. Finally, the cord end was found, re-clamped, tied off and the incision closed. It was only after the surgery was over did Dr. T tell him what had happened. Any sooner and that young man might have jumped off the table and run out of the room. I can think of a few other times I wouldn't want to hear someone say "Oh-Oh". I wouldn't want my barber saying it, the pilot of a plane and certainly not my surgeon. I tried hard not to say it myself during any of the procedures I did.

Early one morning, around 2 am, I received a call from a Georgia State Patrol (GSP) dispatcher requesting my assistance. Apparently, there was an accident on I-20 west of Thomson. A car had been hit by an eighteen wheeler. There were three people killed and one trapped in the car. Those on the scene needed help trying to find a way to extricate the trapped passenger. The dispatcher told me he had called several physicians in the area before Dr. T suggested he call me. I was asleep and didn't know whether the call was legit or not, so before I left, I called back. I had learned my lesson from having rushed to an airplane accident early in my youth. The GSP dispatcher assured me it was for real and I decided to get up and go. How many times does one get a call from the GSP? I left my wife and new baby at home at 2 am headed to a wreck on I-20. What was I getting into?

An eighteen wheeler heading east on I-20 from Atlanta had rounded a curve when the driver saw headlights in front of him. He swerved to the right in order to avoid a head-on collision and drove right up over two cars which were in the emergency lane. Apparently what he saw were the headlights of one car facing another car that people were trying to jump start.

The wreck was over twenty miles from my home and in the middle of nowhere. I put the pedal to the metal, figuring they had called me and headed west. I could see lights ahead which were coming from a large crane that had been brought to the scene. When I got there I saw this horrible scene and smelled diesel fuel everywhere. I slipped on the diesel fuel crossing over to the east bound side. Our county sheriff had driven up to see the accident and yelled at me to watch my step or they might just have to treat me.

I crawled down to the car and spoke to the emergency medical technician (EMT) who had been comforting a trapped lady. The roof and dashboard were collapsed onto her legs, pinning her in the car. I looked up to see the engine and tires of the eighteen wheeler hanging precariously over us. The patient was alert and our greatest fear was what would happen when we took the weight of the dash off her in order to free her. Was the weight of the dash working like a tourniquet and preventing her from bleeding to death? Were her legs even attached?

The EMT and I decided that she couldn't stay in the car much longer and we made the decision to jack the dash up. The roof was already peeled back some by the truck and we could take her out that way. The dash was jacked up, her legs were still attached and the bleeding was minimal. She was taken out through the roof on a back board and later placed on a stretcher. The last time I saw her was when she was placed in an awaiting ambulance and taken to the nearest ER. I had made my first really big decision as a new PA and cemented my role in the area with the local law enforcement.

I remember my first baby delivery very well. While I was gowning-up and putting my gloves on, I placed my right hand into the left glove the nurse was holding for me. Then I placed my left hand into the right glove she was holding. I remembered, when hit with the unexpected, do what you were trained to do. Neither the nurse nor I said anything and a new baby was welcomed into the world.

About this time, a new class of drugs had been released to help heal stomach ulcers and the pain associated with them. A patient had come in who I thought would be a good candidate for the drug. The product was to be prescribed for short term treatment for patients not responding to regular antacid therapy. The patient returned in a month and informed me that this new medicine was a godsend. "I can drink a whole case of beer without hurting now." What had I unleashed by prescribing this new wonder drug for him? I confess, I backed off of prescribing it because I didn't want to create a bigger problem.

Life in a small town was very rewarding. I had met a lot of good people and had developed a close relationship with law enforcement personnel. This came in handy one day when I was heading into town and came up to a GSP check point. I couldn't find my license anywhere. The closer I got to this officer the more anxious I got. When I pulled up to him he recognized me and asked me what I knew about hemorrhoids. I answered what do you want to know and he just waived me on through. He never asked to see my license which I found later in my wallet.

The seven years I spent with Dr. T in Family Practice were some of my best years. Dr. T had taught me a lot of medicine and about life in general. During the seventies our country was going through double digit inflation. Debbie and I were expecting our second daughter and I never received a pay raise. I had delivered a few babies, assisted in surgery and treated some great patients. Despite all this it was time to explore other options.

The pharmaceutical representatives who called on us drove new cars, wore expensive suits and earned good salaries. An opportunity to change direction presented itself and I was off again to another new adventure.

WHERE'S THE PATCH?

I made the decision to become a pharmaceutical representative and applied for an Augusta territory. My background as a Physician Assistant helped me land the job. I had prescribed several of the products the company represented and knew what the job involved.

I went to work for a Fortune 500 company which had a diverse product line. The company sold the number one selling hormone replacement product and the number one selling antihypertensive drug at the time.

I already knew several area physicians from growing up at the hospital and I saw this as a chance to expand my role as a PA. The way I saw it was that every time a physician wrote my product it was like me prescribing it. Over the years, I was promoted to a Regional Trainer and Hospital Representative.

My sales territory included the Central Savannah River Area (CSRA) along with some South Carolina counties. I called on local physicians, hospitals and drug stores mainly. This required some overnight stays which turned out to be adventures all their own.

On one of my first overnights, I was awakened by the pitter-patter of something running in the attic of my room. It sounded like rats running back and forth. I couldn't get back to sleep and finally called the desk clerk. I was told not to worry. It was only squirrels chasing each other. "They come in at night to get out of the cold", the clerk said. He then added, "Have a good night." Sure, I thought, you try sleeping with squirrels running all over your head.

At another motel, I was awakened by something chewing at my bathroom window screen. I looked out and saw deer all over the place. It seems that over the years, motel guest had been feeding deer and attracting them to the motel. Oh, the joys of staying in motels in the rural South!

I was waiting in the reception area of a physician office, in a small town, when a young girl came out. She had just seen the physician and her mother asked her, "What did he tell you was wrong?" The girl answered, "I don't know. I couldn't understand a word he said." Then she added, "But he did give me these prescriptions." The mother replied, "Good." The physician was foreign trained and spoke very little English and I wondered how many patients left his office every day and didn't even know what was wrong with them.

In another office the physician came out and started laughing. He saw me and said, "You've got to hear this". Apparently he had written a competitor's hormone replacement product which came in the form of a patch. Instead of taking a pill daily, the patient only had to apply a patch each month. Well, this patient did as directed and applied a patch each month. She had come in that day with an unexpected problem. She was complaining of not having any more places to apply a patch without it being seen. She added that no one ever told her to take the old patches off. She must have been about two bricks short of a load.

As I mentioned, my territory was rather large and required a lot of travel. Most of my traveling was done on rural back roads. From time to time nature would call when I was in the middle of nowhere. So, I could relate to the following story I heard about another unfortunate person caught off guard.

Apparently something similar happened to a man driving in the country. He found himself having to relieve himself and there were no restrooms around. He turned down a dirt road, got out and began to relieve himself. He was bitten by something on the tip of his thing which began to swell immediately. He was in a great deal of pain and set off to find help. He drove to the nearest country store and went inside, where he was met by two elderly ladies. Without thinking, he whipped out his thing and asked, "What can you give me for this?" The first gal replied, "I'll give you the store and my forty Ford." The second added, "I'll throw in thirty acres of prime bottom land."

I remember one time while calling on a drug store in the town adjacent to Thomson, the following took place. When I entered the drug store, the pharmacist greeted me by name. A customer overheard him and asked me if I was a PA. I said, "Yes" and she replied, "You delivered my baby." Then she added quickly "But, you probably don't recognize me from this position." We all had a good laugh at that.

As my pharmaceutical career progressed, I was promoted to a trainer for new representatives. In addition to covering my sales territory this position required me to fly all over the country. I flew so often that Delta even made me a Flying Colonel. This allowed me to use their Crown Rooms as I traveled to cities like San Francisco, Dallas, Mobile, Atlanta, New York, Chicago, San Antonio and Montreal, Canada.

While teaching a class in San Francisco, I took the students south to Half Moon Bay for dinner. There we saw the great grey whales migrating from Alaska during our meal and one of the most beautiful Pacific sunset I had ever seen.

Not only did we train new reps, we were also trained in the latest sales techniques. We met in Chicago one year for our trainers training meeting. We were introduced to new sales skills being used by companies like IBM and Xerox. We would take these newly acquired skills and teach our new reps. I always felt that being a Trainer was the best position in the company. We were treated like semi-management, given top bonuses and got to visit a lot of cool places.

We went out for dinner in one of Chicago's most famous steak restaurants. The meal consisted of the best house steak, some great wine and was capped off with imported cigars. The total price for the thirteen of us set a new record for any one meal charged to the Training Department.

While in San Antonio we were taken out for dinner on river barges and enjoyed several trips up and down the San Antonio River savoring our a la carte meal. If you haven't realized by now, I really enjoyed eating out.

New representatives spent six months in training before earning the title of Pharmaceutical Representative. The training is broken down into three phases. The first phase was spent in a motel room with a District manager who would review company policy and our product line. The second phase included two weeks in a regional sales office where a trainer, like myself, would review pharmacology, pharmacodynamics and pharmacokinetics of our major products. In other words, we would cover how our drugs worked and were prescribed for use in the treatment of certain diseases like hypertension, epilepsy, migraines and osteoporosis. During phase three, reps from all over the country would converge on Glenn Cove, New York for their last two weeks of formal sales training. Here they were introduced to sales techniques and how to market our products. We would video tape these sessions so they could see how they did using company brochures during staged physician presentations. There would be a graduation party for all the reps where they received a certificate of achievement granting them the title of Pharmaceutical Representative.

At that time, the company was using a conference center in Glenn Cove, on Long Island. Originally, the center was called "The Manor" which was built in 1920 on a thirty-five-acre estate. The center later became known as the Glenn Cove Mansion. It is now known as the Harrison Conference Center. The center was located across from the Russian Consulates' quarters in one of the most picturesque areas of our country. The center had a pub located on the top floor and a wood floor bowling alley in the basement where you had to rack your own pins while playing.

During a heavy snow storm, I went out on the balcony and called Debbie. All of the sudden it started to thunder. It was so loud she could hear it on the other end of the phone. I had never expected to hear thunder in the middle of a snow storm. It was a new experience for this southern boy. I thought the world was coming to an end when I heard thunder lightening, in the snow!

After completing the first year, groups of reps would be taken to Montreal, Canada and then to Rouses Point, New York. This was the frosting on the cake for all those reps completing a year of intense training. Of course, the groups were chaperoned by trainers. We stayed in the Queen Elizabeth Hotel, while in Montreal, near the Saint Lawrence River.

It was in the Queen Elizabeth Hotel that I would eat the best seafood buffet on Thursday night, while looking down at the river. I also watched my first nude TV movie there. I couldn't speak French and there wasn't closed caption, so I just made up my own dialog. Oh Lá Lá! I saw my first dinner theatre in Montreal and shopped at the underground stores. It was a great city to visit a couple of times a year.

Thursday afternoon we would go tour our research facilities. The next morning, we would board a bus for Rouses Point, New York where the company's manufacturing and marketing center was located. Rouses Point is just a couple of miles south of the US/Canadian border. In the afternoon we would then head for the airport in Montreal to return home. I got us across the border several times because I had Jimmy Carter's signature on my Georgia Driver's License (he was President four of these years) and my Southern accent didn't hurt either.

As I mentioned earlier, I was flying all over the country and I remember one flight in particular. I was sitting in a plane on the runway in Atlanta that was bound for Glenn Cove. All the passengers were talking, laughing and preparing for takeoff. We were probably number fourteen in the line. The closer we got to liftoff the quieter the cabin got. Everyone knew that most airplane accidents occurred during takeoff or landing. The Rolls Royce engines powered up and the plane headed down the runway. The massive jet started to vibrate as it lifted off. We began to ascend through clouds when a young girl was overheard asking her mother, "Are we going to heaven now?" Well you could have heard a pin drop as those of us sitting near them awaited the mothers reply. After what seemed like an eternity the mother finally answered, "No. Not now." A sigh of relief came over everyone and we settled on in for the flight.

I often wondered what made physicians prescribe one product over another product for their patients. My ego believed it was because we trained our sales force so well. I decided to do an informal survey of some of my physicians to find an answer. Most of them gave the standard reasons: safety, efficacy, cost and fewest side effects. Others shared more enlightening reasons.

A physician informed me he wrote our particular antibiotic because it was the only red and black capsule on the market and he had graduated from the University of Georgia. Another said he prescribed products for the reps with the best looking legs. Men or women? Hospital interns and residents seemed to prescribe products for the reps who took them out to lunch while other physicians wanted to write what their patients were seeing on TV. All in all, my ego took a big blow.

In very good years, the company would throw a national sales meeting to thank all the employees for their efforts. This was a great time for me because I got to see former trainers, managers and reps I had helped to train. I also knew a lot of the regional managers and could go almost anywhere and be instantly recognized. Even the big wigs knew me from their trips to the graduation ceremonies at Glenn Cove each year. It was hard to keep my ego under check. During one of the evening ceremonies, the trainers were being recognized for our role in the success of the company and our hard work. After being recognized I started to sit down when the chair folded up and I landed on my butt with my chin on the table. Some of those sitting at the table couldn't help it and started to laugh. The speaker even asked over the microphone if I was alright, which drew more attention to what had happened. My ego was shattered and for the rest of the meeting I was called "Grace".

LISTING TO THE RIGHT

I spent twelve and a half years working as a Pharmaceutical Representative, and during the entire time, I had the same District manager. District managers are the watch dogs over the sales force. They fill vacancies, help train new reps, motivate them and oversee the sales in their respective districts. Each manager for our company had about twelve reps that he/she was responsible for. Their main role was making certain that sales goals were met. I had never sold anything, except maybe a few cars, before beginning this journey and my manager had some very helpful tips most of the time.

My manager also had several health issues which plagued him over his entire career. The most notable was flatulence. That's right. He farted a lot. Farting is a very common natural bodily function for most of us. Estimates are that we normally pass gas 10 times a day while respecting those around us. There are a number of causes for flatulence, and I won't attempt to cover them all here, however, some notable causes are swallowing air while drinking or eating too fast. Some foods like beans and cabbage are also known to contribute to the problem along with certain health issues like constipation, irritable bowel syndrome (IBS), celiac disease and gallbladder disease. The latter is what the PA side of me decided was my manager's problem.

Early on, I realized that he had a real problem with gas. We were sitting in a doctor's waiting room when I got my first hint. If you have ever been in a physician's waiting room, you know how quiet it can be. Everyone is sitting around whispering or reading three-year-old magazines to pass the time. Well, it was during just one of these visits when he listed to the right and let out a very audible fart. Everyone started looking around for the culprit and he just sat there expressionless, like nothing had happened. After leaving the office after one of these incidents, I suggested that he have his gallbladder checked out. It didn't just happen in the waiting room.

During sales presentations to physicians, it wasn't unusual for him to start squirming, list to the right and cut one just as I was in midsentence. He would just sit there like a frog on a rock and say nothing. Most physicians would look at me with an expression of disbelief. I would always suggest later that he get his gallbladder checked out. His ability to list to the right and let one fly would come when you least expected it. I would go back the next day and apologize to the physician for him. Most of the physicians would have a good laugh and that was that, especially after they learned I thought it was his gallbladder.

Prior to district meetings several of us would get together and discuss whether this happened to them recently. Many would share similar embarrassing moments when the urge hit him. One thought he was going to fill a balloon during a visit with him. Another thought he could play tunes as long as the range was between B flat and A sharp. We would go to the meetings anticipating when his next bout was going to occur and wait to see if anyone would crack up when he started listing to the right.

I don't want to sound like I'm making fun of what was probably a legitimate medical problem for my manager, however, it seemed to occur at times when least expected and he would never show any emotion or apologize. I believe he could have controlled this because he would telegraph its arrival.

When I became a hospital rep, I would take the stairs whenever he visited. This accomplished several things. First, it would shake lose any gas. Second, it wore him out and Third, I didn't have to be embarrassed in an elevator when he cut one.

I don't know if he ever had his gallbladder checked out or whether his listing to the right had anything to do with testing my ability to be a pharmaceutical representative or not. I only know that it took every ounce of control I/we could muster not to lose it when he began listing to the right.

I enjoyed the years I spent as a pharmaceutical rep and trainer. The down side was I had missed out on a lot of my daughters' school activities and helping Debbie out. I had missed way too many Friday night football games sitting on runways waiting for planes to take off. Heather was in the high school band and Jennifer was a middle school cheerleader. It was time to move on.

A PET FLYING SQUIRREL

I became an Instructor and the Clinical Director at my Alma Mater, The Medical College of Georgia, in 1992. This was a good fit which enabled me to combine my sales experience and territory organizational skills. As Clinical Director my responsibility was to set up clinical rotations for twenty students to attend during the last twelve months of the two-year program. Each student had to spend seven, six-week long rotations in each of the following disciplines: Internal Medicine, Surgery, Family Medicine, Pediatrics, Obstetrics and Gynecology, Emergency Medicine and Mental Health. Rotation sites were located primarily throughout South Carolina and Georgia and provided a vital role in the training of our students. In addition to the clinical rotations they had to spend another six weeks in an Elective like: Dermatology, Cardiology and Family Medicine. All these rotations combined added up to 160 rotations per year that I had to arrange. I even set up two International Electives; one in Venezuela and another in India. I tried really hard to get the school to send me on a site visit in each of these countries, but they never bit.

As part of our Federal Training Grant each student was expected to do at least one of their rotations in a medically underserved area. This was required in an attempt to recruit health care providers into areas where they were most needed. To help make this experience more appealing, several communities provided free housing for the entire six weeks. This also saved students from having to pay for six weeks of lodging out of pocket. In theory, if a student spent six weeks in a community they just might move there after graduation. Physicians might even move into these towns because they wouldn't be the only health care provider in the area.

I received a call from a hospital administrator with an unusual problem. One of our students had shown up for his six-week rotation with his wife, three children, several birds and a pet flying squirrel. The administrator didn't know what to do. He had not expected an entire family to show up. I had to call the student and remind him that the free housing was for him and not intended for his wife, three children, several birds and a pet flying squirrel. Give me a break!

An OB-Gyn called about another student issue. This physician had trained pilots during WWII and had taught our students for years. He wanted to know why I had sent him this particular student. He asked, "What have I done to deserve this student?" Apparently the student thought he knew more than the doctor and constantly second guessed him in front of his patients. He even told him how to perform surgery! The student would not pull call with him as required during rotations and would return home on weekends to wait tables. "I had to tell him to go home because I couldn't teach him anything else." I apologized to the physician and called the student. He confirmed that he had done so well on the rotation that the doctor sent him home. "The doctor told me to go home because he couldn't teach me anything else." This student apparently had an IQ of room temperature and an ego the size of Texas!

My duties as an Instructor consisted of overseeing the Oncology course, holding small group sessions and co-teaching the communication course during the first year. In small groups, students learned how to take a medical history and perform a physical examination. During the communication course they learned how to ask patients questions, assimilate a medical history and prioritize it all into a treatment plan for the patient. Remember, I still had to set up all those clinical rotations for the students who were in the last year of the program.

During the communication course, I would share the following story. A physician once told me that he had been seeing a ninety-year-old patient in the hospital for several weeks. He would go by and see her daily. While reviewing her progress one day, he told her that she would be going home Saturday. She seemed to brighten up and appeared excited about the good news. He went to discharge her that Saturday and learned she had died earlier that morning. I guessed that to her, going home must have meant going to her heavenly home. I would stress to the students that they had to watch what they said because the patients would be hanging onto everything they were told.

Allied Health faculty didn't make a lot of money. In an effort to help bring our salaries up to national averages, we were allowed to start seeing walk-in patients in the Family Practice Center. During one of these visits, I learned the patient I was seeing was a lawyer. After the exam, I told him I thought he might benefit from a prescription. When I returned with his prescription he looked at it and said, "I can't read a thing on this." Without thinking, I replied, "You're not supposed to." Thank goodness he laughed.

One of the attending physicians was well known for wanting to see the color of any nasal secretion from patients complaining of a sinus infection. He would even have the family medicine residents show him nasal samples. This was one way he determined whether the patient had a real sinus infection or not. I had just finished seeing such a patient when he walked into the room to review the case. I had previously obtained a nasal specimen and placed the tissue on top of a waste receptacle. The physician sat down on the receptacle and asked to see any nasal material. I told him he was sitting on it. From that day forward he never asked me if I had any other samples. He even wrote a recommendation letter which helped me get an appointment to Assistant Professor.

It started off like a normal day for me in the Family Practice Center. I was ready to see the walk-in patients when some of the staff noticed I wasn't looking well or acting my usual self. They asked me how I felt and I told them I thought I was just getting over the flu. A check of my pulse and vital signs suggested something else. My heart rate was rapid and irregular. An EKG confirmed I was in atrial fibrillation, ventricular tachycardia and atrial flutter. In simpler terms my heart was beating fast and was not regular. This was not allowing blood to pass through my heart normally and might cause serious blood clots. I was placed in a wheelchair and was directly admitted to the hospital.

When I got to my room one of the cardiologist was at my side within minutes. I was started on an IV with some medication to smooth out my heart. He also began to massage my carotid arteries. These measures successfully converted my heart back into normal sinus rhythm. Immediately I felt like an elephant had been lifted off my chest. I was ready to resume seeing patients but was made to stay in the hospital for heart monitoring. Our daughter Heather, who also worked at MCG, had already called Debbie about my admission. Things happened so quickly that she hadn't arrived from Thomson before I was out of the woods.

By the end of the day I had received flowers from the Family Medicine Department and several PA and FP faculty had visited. I was in a semi-private room and requested a private one. This was my first hospitalization. Dinner was served and I ate a hamburger with some French fries. A short time later I was transferred into the private room I had requested. Another dinner was brought in. The server said, "Here's your dinner, Mr. Jones," and simply left it. This was like being at home because I had two hamburgers with fries for dinner that night. I hope Mr. Jones got something to eat. The rest of the night was uneventful.

The next morning my attending physician came to see how I was doing. I wanted her to discharge me because I had a lot of student responsibilities. She reluctantly agreed to discharge me and setup some outpatient follow up appointments for additional studies. This only happened after a lot of pleading and promises on my part to be a good boy. I will always be thankful for her listening to me, the patient. Maybe she had heard I taught the communication course and stressed the importance of listening to the patient. I was put on Warfarin (a blood thinner) which I learned to hate because of all the PT/INR blood testing that would follow. I went home and prepared for students and patients again.

An elderly man came into the Family Practice Center without an appointment. I got to see him because he was a walk-in. He only wanted a refill of his male enhancement drug. I asked him how many he needed, because I knew they cost about six dollars each. He appeared to be in his mid-eighties and paused before answering, "Six. I break them in half so six should last about a month." I said, "Excuse me, you want six?" What a blessed man he must be I thought. I even entertained becoming a sales rep again just to market this product.

Some of us spent vacation time performing employee physicals at various petroleum companies located throughout the southeast. A van would go to a refinery a couple of weeks ahead of us and collect medical information from the employees. This information included a health history, lab tests, EKG and audio testing. We would then follow-up and perform a hands on OSHA physical. We also reviewed the previously collected information with each employee and if we found any abnormalities she/he would be referred to a local physician for follow-up. All our expenses were paid along with a very good weekly salary.

During one of the examinations, I was proceeding to perform a prostate exam. I asked the employee to place his elbows on the exam table and assume the proper position. While I was inserting my finger, a very loud squeal came out of my glove as some trapped air leaked out. He clamped down on my finger so hard that I almost couldn't get it out. I tried not to laugh, or wiggle my finger and we just acted like nothing had happened.

After completing a long day of OSHA physicals, I went out on the balcony of the condo room the company had rented while I was in Port Author, Texas. Port Author is located below Beaumont on the Intercoastal Water Way and very close to the Gulf of Mexico. The condo was located in a marina and I was sipping on a cold beer listening to the bells ringing atop the masts of several sailboats berthed there. I was talking to Debbie on the phone when a flock of large pink birds came flying over. I told her this and she wanted to know how many beers had I had. I assured her I wasn't kidding and that there were maybe thirty or forty large pink birds flying over the marina. Well Debbie, who knows everything, knew right away what they were. She told me they were flamingos flying to some place nearby. I didn't even know flamingos flew and felt like Jethro Bodine in the Beverly Hillbillies. Heck sake, up until that very moment, I had only seen flamingos standing in people's front yards. This is the kind of education you don't get in college.

Doing OSHA petroleum physicals allowed me to visit other places like a mesa in Big Spring, Texas, the Carville Leprosarium in Carville, Louisiana and eating crawfish in Rayne, Louisiana.

Anyone who has had Leprosy (now known as Hansen's disease) probably knows about the National Leprosarium located in Carville, Louisiana. To my knowledge everyone needing in house treatment went to Carville. The campus is located off a two lane highway in Southern Louisiana and very near the Mississippi River. I drove down that two lane highway, which followed a levee for miles until I found the Leprosarium. The campus was very large and shaded by sprawling Live Oaks covered in moss.

Cottages were scattered about and were mostly two story, white structures that were in need of repair. Row crops were planted at the edges of the campus which was located on what was once a sugar plantation. It looked kind of grown up and spooky and I wondered what it sounded like at night with all the river critters. I learned later that the Leprosarium was going to move and that only a few longtime residents were going to stay.

I drove a few more miles down the river road and found a cut through the levee and a cable drawn barge used to ferry the river. It was as close to what I imagined the Huck Finn days were like. Time appeared to be standing still.

By now the PA program was accepting forty students per year. This meant I had to set up 320 clinical rotations per year in addition to my first year student responsibilities. Teaching had been great but seeing patients again in the Family Practice Center reminded me of how much I really enjoyed being a health care provider. I started searching for something new.

TOO MANY SHOWERS

I missed treating patients and went to work at the Augusta Youth Detention Center (YDC). The facility is run by the Department of Juvenile Justice (DJJ) and houses many of our state's mentally challenged youth offenders. My past experiences as an ambulance attendant, ER orderly and Vietnam corpsman were all put to the test during this journey.

The YDC is located on Highway 56 across from the old Proctor and Gamble plant. It was a forty-five-mile trip from Thomson, one way. I would take I-20 to I-520 to Highway 56 south. I had plenty of time during the commute to listen to the radio. Debbie doesn't appreciate country music so I used this time to listen to it regularly. A new song had come out about a guy who went one round, two rounds, even ten rounds with another guy named José Cuervo. I never really knew why he continued going round after round with José. I figured José was either a boxer from South America, a shadow boxer or a cage fighter from up North someplace. I liked the beat mainly and enjoyed singing along with it. One day I asked Debbie, because she knows everything, "Who is José Cuervo?" She replied, "José Cuervo isn't a person. It's a brand of tequila." Well, this explained why this guy kept going back for round after round with José. She made me feel like Jethro Bodine again, but I still give the song a ten for its' beat.

I was called to the Detention Unit on my first day at the YDC because a resident had cut himself. I entered the cell and saw blood everywhere. He had put a tourniquet on his arm, cut it and sprayed blood everywhere. He claimed to be an Indian Chief and didn't want to be locked up like this. After several stitches, he was returned to his cell good as new. I tried for years to convince him that an Indian Chief wouldn't cut himself. The braves would look at that as a sign of weakness, not strength (dumb in other words). He wouldn't listen to me and seemed to be about two stories higher than a seven story building.

Walking past the woodshop one morning, I overheard a group of residents talking about their things. One of them saw me and asked what the average size a thing should be. I told him I had always heard it was one-half your shoe size. Before the day was over, I had received several sick call requests from one of our more challenged residents. By the next morning, he had put in several more requests wanting to see me about "a personal matter". I saw him later that morning and all he wanted to know was if he should measure himself hard or soft.

This all male campus only allowed one fifteen-minute shower per day. Like most adolescents, these residents could find a reason to take more frequent and longer showers. They often filled out sick call requests for blood coming out of their thing. A nurse had told one of them that over using their thing could break it and blood might sure enough come out. This spread like wildfire throughout the campus.

I was called another time to check on a resident having what the guards thought was a seizure. I found him lying on a dormitory floor jerking. After examining him, I told the guards it didn't look like a seizure because his left hand wasn't jerking. Guess what? His left hand started to jerk. Residents were always looking for ways to get off campus and having a seizure was just one way. Others would cut themselves or complain of having a dislocated shoulder. I became very accomplished at suturing, stapling and even gluing wounds closed. I even had a few tricks up my sleeve when it came to diagnosing dislocated shoulders.

If a resident came in complaining of a dislocated shoulder I often instructed him to follow my finger, using his good arm, through a series of range of motion exercises. I would suddenly tell him to switch arms and continue to follow my finger. Without blinking an eye most would switch from the good arm to the hurting arm without missing a beat. Most of the residents couldn't think of but one thing at a time, and misdirection cost several of them a trip off campus.

Youth Development Campuses throughout the nation are like small cities. They all provide residents with the basics to sustain life; food, clothing, shelter while serving their sentences. They are also provided health and dental care. Most provide schooling through the twelfth grade and residents can work on a GED/HS diploma. Guards tell residents when to get up, when to shower, when to eat, when to play, when to attend school and when to sleep. Everyone marches in columns to and from activities. Families can only visit on the weekends and only then if their child had been good. Most days are so structured that they didn't allow residents to think on their own.

One resident in particular has stuck with me for years. His name doesn't matter. What does matter was he had been sentenced at age eight to eleven years in the DJJ. The reason for his sentence must have been horrendous. I never knew what he had been sentenced for because I made it a point to never know what any resident's sentence was for. The resident's health was more important. I had the opportunity to walk around campus with him and learn firsthand just how unprepared he was for life outside the system.

He had no work history, never had a date with a girl and didn't even know how to drive a car. He had no clue what Walmart was, or that there was a McDonald's on almost every corner. He didn't know how to apply for a job or even what he wanted to be. I believe he did obtain a high school diploma during his eleven-year sentence and had become a pretty good carpenter. But how was he going to succeed on the outside?

I tried to see what was available for him after his release and couldn't find much. He was going to be released into the real world soon and it appeared he had been set up for failure. Maybe his high school diploma and carpentry experience would be enough to give him a jump start. I just prayed his next stop wouldn't be the state prison system.

I have a great deal of respect for all the employees who work in DJJ facilities. This is a seemingly thankless job yet they are all trying to help the residents survive from day to day.

His name doesn't matter, what does matter is whether he was prepared to meet a world outside the YDC or not. I do know he was in good health and a pleasant young man so I tried to steer him into a health care field.

During this time frame, my heart arrhythmias never really resolved and I spent several years in and out of specialists' offices. I was convinced it was a flavor enhancer known as monosodium glutamate (MSG) that was causing all my problems. Some specialist thought it was my thyroid, still others thought it was stress. I even had my thyroid chemically ablated in an attempt to smooth the heart out. The procedure didn't work out as hoped and Debbie spent many hours reviewing product ingredients for MSG. She began to cook soup and other meals from scratch because almost anything sold in a can contained MSG. When we ate out, I asked the waitress if the food was prepared using MSG. You would laugh at the many times waitresses thought I was trying to pull their legs. Today MSG has been taken out of most processed foods and snacks because of its association to arrhythmias, allergies and migraines. Most restaurants have even backed off using it and now list their meals as MSG free.

I eventually had to undergo cardiac ablation. During this procedure a catheter is placed in a leg vein, near the groin, and fed up into the heart. A laser beam is sent through the catheter and literally fries any ectopic complexes that are prematurely firing, thus causing the arrhythmias. Every time an impulse hits along the heart's conductive system, the heart muscles contract forcing blood through the heart and into the body. If the arrhythmias go on uncontrolled a blood clot could develop and then it could become life threatening. The procedure was done at University Hospital and everything went along smoothly. I tried to be a good patient.

The time came when I was able to combine my YDC and MCG years and retire early from state employment. My next adventure was about to begin.

WHERE'S THE PHONE?

This adventure grew out of my previous employment at the YDC. The Medical Director for the facility learned I was going to retire early, and he wanted to know if I would help him increase his nursing home practice. This would be a perfect part-time business which I could grow if I wanted to. I had now gone full circle in all my years as a health care provider. You might even say I had treated patients from the cradle to the grave.

During the admission process to a nursing home I often included the following statement to a new resident. "You are in an excellent facility. The nurses can handle about ninety percent of your daily needs, if you tell them. If they can't handle them, they will call the doctor or me with the remaining ten percent. If we can't handle it, we will take you out back and shoot you." I couldn't begin to tell you how many patients responded with laughter. Some even added it was the first time they had laughed since being in the hospital. That one simple statement seemed to set the stage for a speedy recovery. It might even, subconsciously, have set the stage for this writing because laughter can have healing properties.

I found myself seeing the parents and grandparents of high school classmates. I even saw neighbors and fellow church members over the years. Toward the end of this journey I was starting to see classmates, which became a reality check for me.

I will never forget one patient who I learned later had been a nurse at University Hospital. She remembered watching me grow up beside the hospital. She recalled seeing me washing the cars, playing in the fish pond, shooting hoops and just being a kid. She turned out to be the mother of one of my fellow church members. The daughter shared the following with me after her mother's death.

"When mother learned who you were she knew she was in good hands and that it was time to give up the fight. She knew everything was going to be alright and that she had nothing but good memories." She added her mother looked so at ease and told her she didn't want to continue being in and out of hospitals anymore. The daughter thanked me for being one of her mother's health care providers. This really shook me up at first.

On a lighter side, a nurse told me that one day a patient's phone was missing and everyone was running around in a panic trying to find it. Suddenly it dawned on the nurse to have the daughter call her father's phone. They heard it ringing in the next room. The patient admitted he had taken it and had hidden it in his pajama bottoms. The nurse later told him not to take any more phones and if he did, the least he should do would be to put it on the vibration mode. That way it couldn't be heard and he just might get a thrill.

I first met Robert in one of my nursing homes early on during this journey. He was sitting in his wheelchair beside a bird cage in the day room. This was his usual place in the mornings. Robert suffered from a type of disability that affected his body movement and posture. The disability was related to problems associated with brain development most likely. He had been confined to a wheelchair and bed most of his life. He communicated with people by smiling, blinking his eyes or making grunting gestures.

Robert enjoyed McDonald hamburgers, cokes and an occasional beer. His condition gradually worsened over time. His body became more constricted and he began to aspirate food. He eventually became a high-risk patient for solid food aspiration which could lead to pneumonia. He was started on liquid shakes and pureed food. Despite continued medical intervention he continued to decline until becoming totally bed bound and less interactive with stuff. He was in and out of the hospital with aspiration related problems. His family requested he have a feeding tube. Despite all this Robert never really complained. He would continue to let his needs be known by smiling, winking or grunting. This went on for several years until one night while the nursing assistants were bathing him they noticed a dramatic change. Robert's extremities were not as stiff or contracted as usual. His faced looked much more relaxed and he was smiling more. It was as if he was changing into a new person right in front of them. He became more interactive and appeared less stressed out. Robert died the next morning, free of constricted limbs and apparently a new man. Most of the staff knew they had witnessed a miracle.

My mother-in-law, Connie, also became a patient. She was in her mid-seventies when she was admitted to Trinity Hospital for hip surgery. She had always been active and traveled several times abroad with her husband Allan.

They had seen the Swiss Alps, Italy, London and most of Europe. They had a passion for golf and were members of the Augusta Country Club. Allan and I rarely beat her at golf because she stayed in the middle of the fairway, while we played from the rough. She and Allan were enjoying the good life until his unexpected death at age sixty-three. For almost twenty years she took care of herself and lived independently for as long as she could. Connie's last sister-in-law had died about six months before her hip fracture. At the grave side services, Debbie and I noticed she didn't look well. She had lost weight, slowed down and was using a cane for balance. We knew she had had breast cancer surgery and was just probably not feeling well.

During hip surgery the physicians found she had bone cancer. This is one of the most debilitating and painful of cancers. It carried a very poor prognosis. The Connie we knew, who had managed her own affairs now needed some help. She asked me what I thought about her prognosis for recovery. I asked her what she wanted to do and explained all her options. We then set up an appointment with my supervising physician who would go over her options again.

The family met in his office and videotaped the session. The bone cancer had already metastasized (spread) through her body by the time the hip fracture occurred. It didn't look good and she knew it. She asked how much time she would have with treatment and without treatment. We told her only God knew. She kept pressing us until we finally gave her our best estimate, maybe a year with treatment and six months without. She opted out of treatment and we all agreed that she would be as comfortable as possible during her remaining time. This lady took only Extra Strength Tylenol for pain up until she entered hospice. She remained independent to a fault at times. I remember her asking me once if she was ahead of schedule or on schedule. I answered ahead and she responded with her usual wit, "Well aren't you a bright ray of sunshine." I think it was her way of thanking me for being straight forward with her.

We were all at her home for her birthday. We had good fellowship reminiscing about her life and watching her play with her great grandson Brenton. She ate some birthday cake before retiring for the evening. I went into her room before leaving for Thomson and apologized to her for not having told Allan and her earlier how much I appreciated them accepting me into the family. I wanted to let her know how much I loved her and told her to tell Allan the same. In fact, I even asked her to tell my mother and father the same when she saw them. She was a strong lady and seemed at peace. Around two in the morning, Debbie and I received a call from the hospice nurse, "Connie has died." What a beautiful life she had had for seventy-seven years. I'm certain she and Allan are playing golf right now.

I experienced some right lower quadrant abdominal pain one night which didn't respond to analgesics. I knew it wasn't my appendix and figured it would just go away. By morning I was in so much pain that I called my supervising physician who wanted to see me immediately. He told me it didn't appear to be appendicitis either but called a surgeon friend of his anyway. I went straight down to be seen by the surgeon who decided to send me to University Hospital for some radiologic studies. He wasn't sure what was causing me so much pain either. The studies suggested diverticulitis and I was admitted for three days of IV antibiotics. During this time several family members came by to brighten my day. I just wish they had brought me a good book to read. Something short and funny maybe. By the fourth day I was good as new and ready to see nursing home patients again.

I had a follow-up colonoscopy scheduled for six months after the bout of diverticulitis. For many years I had recommended screening colonoscopies and had heard all the horror stories. I wasn't without some reservations myself as I prepared for this test. Thank goodness I didn't have to drink all those preparation formulas and only had to take a few pills. I also fasted two days prior to the test. In the wee hours of the day before the test date, around 2am, I awoke with indigestion. I got up, went out to the kitchen, and took some antacids from a blister pack. Later that morning, while at work, Debbie called me. She wanted to know if I had taken anything during the night. I let her know about the antacids and she let me know about the empty blister pack she found for our dog's heart worm medicine. I told her I was feeling fine, but out of an abundance of caution she called our pharmacist to see if there might be side effects I would need to watch out for. She even called our veterinarian and told him what I had done. She had to add, "And he is a Physician Assistant". Both the pharmacist and vet had a good laugh. After reassurance from both of them, she called to share the good news with me. The next morning, I went for my colonoscopy and told the physician what I had done informing him that "I should be clean as a whistle and free of heart worms, too!". I believe this was a first for him because he started to laugh to the point of tears. This kind of put a new meaning to the warning, "Keep medicine out of the reach of children".

A nursing home admission director came up to me one morning wanting to see if we would take a new patient. This patient had requested a change in providers and she thought of us. He had been a chaplain during WWII and was in the nursing home for rehab. He had served in the South Pacific during some of the worst battles and had been severely burned. His current physician would not order him a nightly scotch and water, so he wanted to change providers. I always tried to make the nursing home experience as stressless as possible and if a resident usually had a beer, glass of wine, or a scotch and water in the evening, why not. He didn't have any health issues to deny the request, so we accepted him. He became a more pleasant patient during the rest of his stay.

Working in nursing homes required a lot of walking. I always tried to wear name brand comfortable shoes. I started having left heel pain one month which seemed to be getting worse. My shoes had air pockets in the heels, which were supposed to absorb shock. I began to notice a kind of crunching, clicking sound coming from my shoes. This progressed to the point that I couldn't wear the shoes without pain or crunching. I asked Debbie, because she knows everything, to check them out. She looked at the heels and found a small tear in the left one. It appeared that over time small stones/pellets had begun to fill up one of the air chambers. This was causing the crunching, clicking sound and making my left heel hurt. Debbie widened the tear, emptied the stones and filled the chamber with glue. The shoes became wearable again and didn't make a sound. I can't begin to think of what the nurses were thinking as I crunched and clicked my way down the halls.

Now that I have retired, Debbie and I are camping more. On one trip, I met a retired dentist who had served during the Vietnam era. He also had called on nursing homes, while in private practice, and he shared the following with me. "On one of my visits I entered a resident's room and introduced myself to the ladies inside. I saw a bowl of peanuts on a nearby table. I started to eat some of them and noticed the ladies began looking strangely at one another. I apologized for not asking them first if I could have some peanuts. They replied, "Oh that's ok. We don't like peanuts and just suck the chocolate off them and put them back into that bowl." He told me he began to choke and never assumed anything after that.

Well, I guess everybody has some memories or tales they could share and I hope you have enjoyed laughing at a few of mine. Everyone at one time or another should be a half bubble out of plumb, so go ahead and make somebody laugh today. I'm already looking forward to my next adventure. Maybe I'll write a book.

ACKNOWLEDGEMENT

I need to recognize the hundreds of health care providers that I have met and worked with next to fifty years. I was surrounded by the best and trusted each of them in their respected roles. Kudos to those in housekeeping who realized that a clean facility promotes good health while an unclean facility tends to close. I tried to thank each one I came in contact with because they are on the front lines fighting infections. The Dieticians who recognize that a full recovery begins with a well-nourished full belly. The Certified Nursing Assistants (CNA's) who recognize that a clean patient is a healthy patient. They were my eyes and ears recognizing skin lesions/mental changes in patients and letting me know. Thanks goes out to all the Registered Nurses, Physical Therapists, Occupational Therapists, Pharmacists and Physician Assistants I met along the way. I have respected their individual roles in a team approach to medicine. We all worked under the premise of first do no harm and when in doubt ship them out for advanced care. God blessed me with the ability to recognize and treat a number of health care needs while surrounding me with vast numbers of great health care providers. He showed me early on that humor combined with the ability to laugh and make someone else laugh is one way to speed up the healing process. Last, but not least, a special thanks to all my supervising and non-supervising physicians who trusted in me while supporting my role in the delivery of health care.

ABOUT THE AUTHOR

Born in Pennsylvania and educated in Georgia. Winston H. Hunt, PA received his Bachelor of Science degree from the school of Allied Health Sciences at the Medical College of Georgia in Augusta, Georgia. He later became the Director and Assistant Professor in the Program.

Through his medical career, he has worked as an ambulance attendant, emergency room and nursing home orderly, U.S. Navy Corpsmen having served in Vietnam and both clinically and academically as a Physician Assistant.

LIST OF PUBLICATIONS

W. Hunt, *Clinician Reviews*, Vol. 9, No. 2, pg. 163-164, For Clinicians Who Would Be Educators, Feb. 1999.

W. Hunt, E. Huechtker, C. Lewis, L. Lee, *Clinical Medicine 2nd Edition*, The Physician Assistant, Interacting with Other Health Care Professionals, pg. 62, 1996. (textbook)

W. Hunt, *Experience: International Style*, Allied Health – Graduate & Professional Issue, pg. 40-41, Fall/Winter 1994.

L. Lee, C. Lewis, W. Hunt, *Healthcare Assistance*, Allied Health – Graduate and Professional Issue, pg. 12 & 19, 1993-1994 edition.

W. Hunt, *Country Learning*, Allied Health – Minorities Issue, pg. 42-43, Spring 1994.